Fatma Rekik
Faten Frikha
Zouhir Bahloul

Adult celiac disease and associated autoimmune diseases

AF387931

Fatma Rekik
Faten Frikha
Zouhir Bahloul

Adult celiac disease and associated autoimmune diseases

ScienciaScripts

Imprint
Any brand names and product names mentioned in this book are subject to trademark, brand or patent protection and are trademarks or registered trademarks of their respective holders. The use of brand names, product names, common names, trade names, product descriptions etc. even without a particular marking in this work is in no way to be construed to mean that such names may be regarded as unrestricted in respect of trademark and brand protection legislation and could thus be used by anyone.

Cover image: www.ingimage.com

This book is a translation from the original published under ISBN 978-613-9-51621-6.

Publisher:
Sciencia Scripts
is a trademark of
Dodo Books Indian Ocean Ltd. and OmniScriptum S.R.L publishing group

120 High Road, East Finchley, London, N2 9ED, United Kingdom
Str. Armeneasca 28/1, office 1, Chisinau MD-2012, Republic of Moldova, Europe
Printed at: see last page
ISBN: 978-620-4-44901-2

Table of contents

1. Introduction

Celiac disease (CD) is an autoimmune inflammatory enteropathy, caused by one of the protein fractions of gluten (food antigen), gliadin (a protein contained in wheat, rye and barley) and which occurs in genetically predisposed subjects [1,2,3]. Its pathogenesis results from the interaction between genetic, immunological and environmental factors which, through the intervention of the human leukocyte antigen (HLA) class II gene molecules (encoding the HLA-DQ2 molecule, and those encoding the HLA-DQ8 molecule) induce an immune response in the intestinal mucosa leading to villous atrophy resulting in malabsorption, and the presence of specific antibodies in the serum of patients, which have changed the epidemiological view of celiac disease. The heterogeneity of the clinical presentation of CD, ranging from so-called classical forms to frustrated and atypical forms, as well as the existence of totally asymptomatic forms, explain why many cases remain undiagnosed to this day [4]. The association with other autoimmune diseases (AIDs) is frequent, which makes it necessary to systematically search for them.

The aim of our work was to evaluate the prevalence of autoimmune diseases during celiac disease and to analyze their epidemiological, clinical, and immunological profile.

2. Patients and methods

In a retrospective study about 43 cases of celiac disease collected in the internal medicine department of Sfax (between 2000 and 2018), we studied patients with one or more associated autoimmune diseases.

2.1. Patients

❖ In our study, the hospital registry of the internal medicine department was used to identify patients with celiac disease hospitalized between January 2000 and September 2018.

2.1.1.   Inclusion criteria

Patients with celiac disease older than 16 years and with associated autoimmune disease were included.

❖ The diagnosis of celiac disease was made on a combination of clinical, endoscopic, immunologic, histologic, and evolutionary grounds. It is confirmed by intestinal biopsy, which shows total or subtotal villous atrophy (Marsh grades 2 or 3), associated with crypt hyperplasia and increased intraepithelial lymphocytes (greater than 40%) [5].

2.1.2.   Non-inclusion criteria

❖   Under 16 years old

❖ Uncertain diagnosis of celiac disease: negative serology or absence of villous atrophy

❖ Uncertain diagnosis of associated autoimmune disease.

2.2 Methods

2.2.1. *Data collection*

For each patient, we established a canvas with different parameters:

❖ Demographic and clinical data: age, gender

❖ an immunological check-up with research of autoantibodies of celiac disease: anti-transglutaminase (ATG), anti-endomysium (AEM) and research of anti-nuclear antibodies (AAN) and rheumatoid factor (RF)...

❖ The results of the digestive fibroscopy and duodenal biopsy

2.2.2. *Statistical analysis*

All data were entered and analyzed using the *Statistical Package for the Social Sciences* SPSS version 20.0 and Excel.

- *Descriptive study:* We calculated simple frequencies and relative frequencies (percentages) for the qualitative variables. We calculated means, medians and standard deviations (standard derivation) and determined the study of extreme values (minimum and maximum) for quantitative variables.

- ***Analytical study:*** Comparison of means was performed using Student's t-test for independent patient groups or samples (n=2). The significance level retained was $p < 0.05$.

3. Results

3.1- characteristics of patients with autoimmune disease associated with celiac disease

> Among 13,194 patients hospitalized in the internal medicine department during the study period from January 2000 to September 2018, 43 cases of celiac disease were collected, representing a prevalence of 0.32% and an incidence of 2.26 cases per year. The mean age for diagnosis in adulthood was 29 years ±10.33 with extremes ranging from 17 to 65 years.

> Associations with other pathologies were found in 18 patients (41.8%). Their mean age was 29.11 years with extremes ranging from 19 to 47 years.

IAD was diagnosed before CD in 6 patients (33%), concomitantly with CD in 7 patients (38.8%) and after CAM in 5 patients (27.7%). At least 2 diseases were associated with CD in 10 cases (23.2%) and 3 diseases in 2 cases (4.6%) (Table I).

These MAIs were mainly:

> Type 1 diabetes was found in 4 cases (9.3%).

> Other autoimmune conditions were represented by:

- Hypothyroidism in 5 cases or 11.6% while hyperthyroidism was reported in only 1 case. Thyroiditis with positive anti-thyroid antibodies in 4 cases or 9.3%.

- 1 case of autoimmune hepatitis

-   rheumatoid arthritis (RA) in 2 cases (4.6%)

-   Sjögren's syndrome in 3 cases (6.9%), associated with systemic lupus erythematosus (SLE) in 2 cases.

-   SLE was found in 3 cases (6.9%).

-   Antiphospholipid syndrome (APS) in a single case associated with SLE.

-   2 cases of immunological thrombocytopenic purpura (4.6%)

-   Vitiligo associated with periodic disease was genetically confirmed in one patient. Cutaneous psoriasis was diagnosed concomitantly with celiac disease in one patient and hypoparathyroidism was found in 1 case.

-   IgA deficiency was found in 3 cases (6.9%), isolated in one case and part of hypogammaglobulinemia in the other cases.

Table I: Different associated diseases in our patients with celiac disease

Associated diseases	Number of cases	Percentage (%)
Diabetes type 1	4	9,3
Hypothyroidism	5	H,6
Hyperthyroidism	1	2,3
Autoimmune hepatitis	1	2,3
Rheumatoid arthritis	2	4,6
Systemic lupus erythematosus	3	6,9
Sjôgren's syndrome	3	6,9
Antiphospholipid syndrome associated with SLE	1	2,3
Immunologic thrombocytopenic purpura	2	4,6
Vitiligo and periodic disease	1	2,3
Skin Psoriasis	1	2,3
Hypoparathyroidism	1	2,3
IgA deficiency	3	6,8

❖ NAAs, sought in 33 patients in our CD series, were positive in 13 patients (rate >1/160). This NAA positivity was related to a CD-associated connectivitis in 4 cases (SLE associated with Sjögren's syndrome in 2 cases, isolated SLE in 1 case, isolated Sjögren's syndrome in 1 case) and autoimmune thyroiditis in 2 cases with low levels (Table II). In 4 patients with positive NAA, no associated disease was found.

Table II: Summary table of the 6 patients with celiac disease-associated connective tissue disease

Patient n°	Age (years)	Gender	Associated connectivity	Signs of CD	Signs of connectivity	Treatment	Evolution
1	24	female	Rheumatoid arthritis	Weight loss Iron deficiency anemia hypocholesterolemia	Chronic bilateral and symmetrical polyathritis of the large and small joints + synovitis + carpitis stage 3 on hand x-ray	NSAIDs as needed COTANCYL 5mg/d MTX lOmg/week	Correction of anemia then lost sight of
2	35	female	Rheumatoid arthritis	Severe anemia at 4, 5 g/dl Hypocalcemia Hypoalbum inemia Hypocholesterolemia	Chronic bilateral and symmetrical polyarthritis of the large and small joints Carp geodes EN>1000 Anti-CCP positive	In 2015: 3 mini boluses of Methylprednisolone lOOmg/d for 3 days followed by corticosteroid therapy at a dose of 1 Omg/d (MTX CI cytolysis and cholestasis with negative investigation, PBH refused) In 2017: MTX and NSAIDs after spontaneous correction of liver function	Hb ll,4g/dl Normal blood calcium
3	26	female	Systemic lupus erythematosus	Staturo-ponderal delay Delayed puberty Episodes of diarrhea Iron deficiency anemia	Photosensitivity Inflammatory polyarthralgias with arthritis Polyclonal hypergamm aglobulinemia AAN positive at 1/1280	plaquénil	
4	28	female	Systemic	Diarrhea	Weight loss	Plaquenil 200mg 1	Good

			lupus erythematosus and associated Sjögren's syndrome		Skin lesions Oligoarthritis of both ankles Leuc olym phopenia AAN positive at 1/1280 Occular and oral dryness SSA+ SSB Tubular acidosis	cp/d Bicarbonate Kcl lep *3/d	evolution Control endoscopy: normal Anapath: LEL
5	43	female	Systemic lupus erythematosus and associated Sjögren's syndrome	Diarrhea	AAN positive at 1/1280 Occular and oral dryness with SSA+ SSB SAPL	3 boluses of Methylprednisolone followed by high-dose corticosteroid therapy for 6 weeks and then tapering off	Disappearance of anemia
6	20	female	Sjögren's syndrome	Iron deficiency anemia Weight loss Osteomalacia	Occular and oral dryness KPS at the ophthalmic examination Schicholm stage 4 at labial biopsy Bicytopenia Bilateral interstitial Sd Distal tubular acidosis AAN 1/640 SSA+ SSB+ (IN FRENCH)	CTFD for 6 weeks then degression to 2cp of cortancyl	

MTX: methotrexate; KPS: superficial punctate keratitis; CTFD: high dose corticosteroid therapy

OBSERVATION 1

Patient H.W, 35 years old, who was hospitalized for a polyarthritis evolving for 1 year associated with a significant weight loss.

In her history, she had a chronic anemia that had been evolving for 12 years, for which she was followed up in the hematology department, transfused several times and put on martial therapy and folates.

Her history dates back 1 year marked by the onset of anorexia, weight loss and inflammatory arthralgias affecting large and small joints with episodes of arthritis not improved by non-steroidal anti-inflammatory drugs (NSAIDs).

On examination, there was no evidence of chronic diarrhea or skin lesions of psoriasis.

On clinical examination, the patient was thin and pale. There was bilateral and symmetrical polyarthritis: synovitis of both wrists, metacarpophalangeal (MCP) and proximal interphalangeal (IPP) joints, limitation of both shoulders, flessum of both elbows, and pain with limitation of both hips and both knees with positive patellar impingement and metatarsophalangeal (MTP) joint pain.

The biology showed an inflammatory syndrome: sedimentation rate (SV) at 114 mm at 1ère hour and c-reactive protein (CRP) at 153 mg/l, iron deficiency anemia at 4.5 g/dl, hepatic cytolysis at 6 times normal with cholestasis at 2 times normal. HBV and

HCV serologies were negative. Anti-mitochondrial and anti-smooth muscle antibodies were negative.

There was also hypocalcemia with a corrected serum calcium level of 2.1 mmol/L and hypoalbuminemia of 28 g/L. Thyroid stimulating hormone (TSH) was low at 0.01 IU/L.

Immunological investigations showed a strong positive rheumatoid factor (RF) at 181 and then >1000 U/ml, positive anti-citrullinated peptide antibodies (anti-CCP) at 30.5U/ml, positive anti-transglutaminase IgA at 32.5U/ml. Anti-thyroperoxidase (TPO) and anti-R- TSH antibodies were also positive. Anti-nuclear antibodies (ANA) were negative.

<u>Radiologically</u>:

On hand radiography: bilateral stage 3 carpitis with geodes and destruction of the MCP and PPI (Figure 1)

On foot X-ray: geodic images of the MTPs (Figure 2)

On radiography of the pelvis: bilateral coxitis (Figure 3).

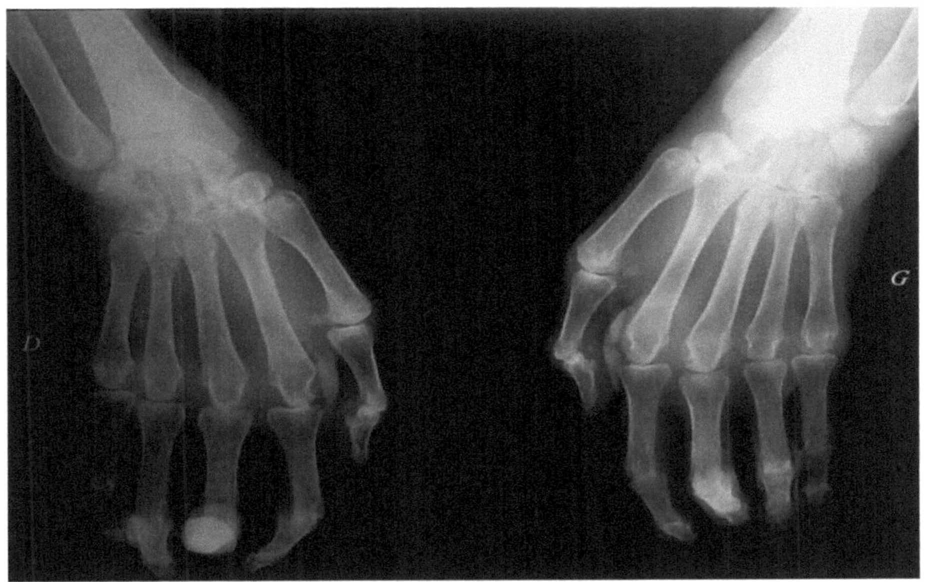

Figure n°1 : X-ray of the hands face: radiocarpal pinch with bilateral carpal tunnel and erosions of the MCP and the IPP

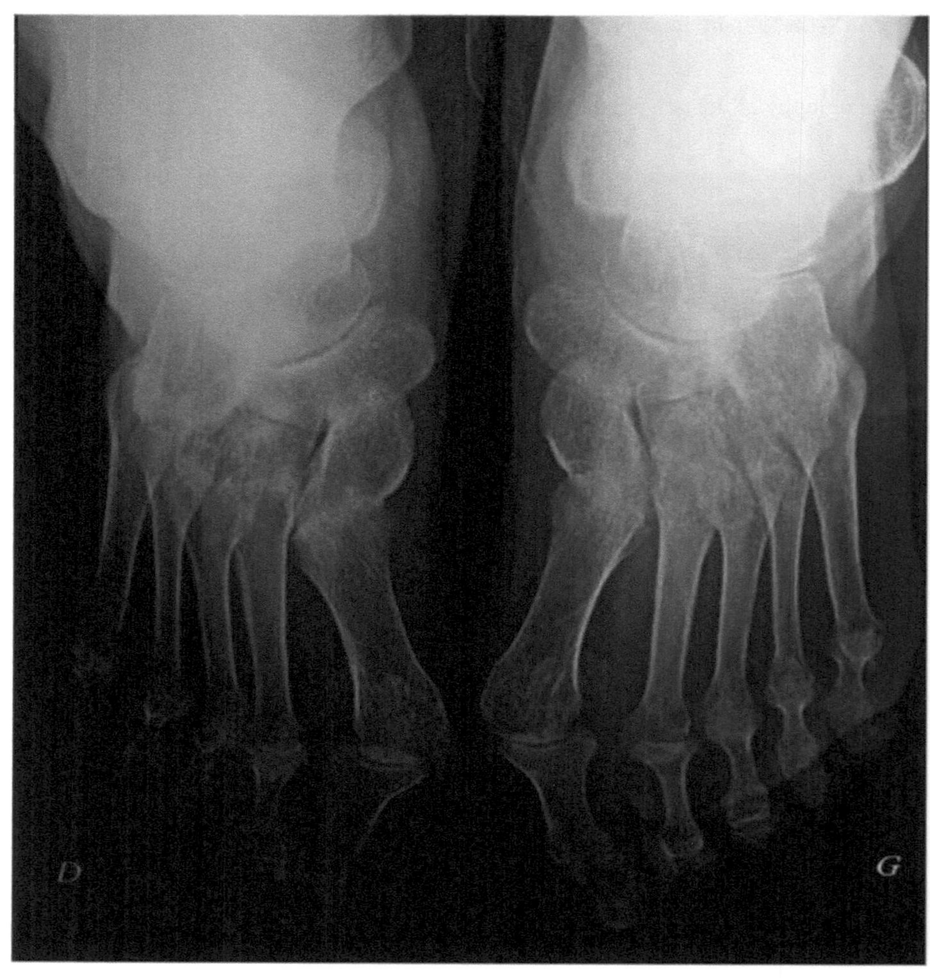

Figure n°2 : X-ray of the feet face : geodic images of the MTP with destruction of

the 2 feet

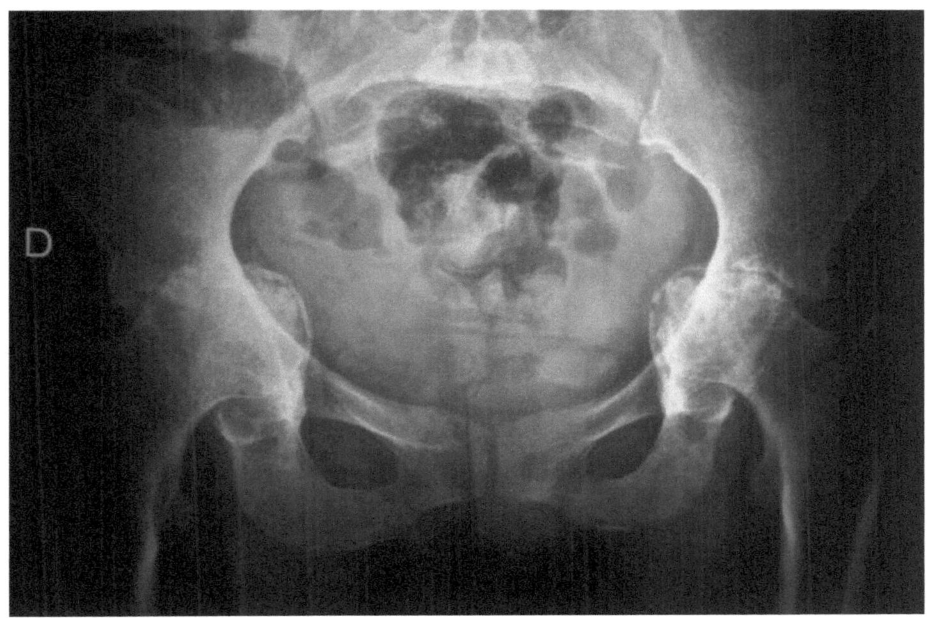

Figure 3: X-ray of the pelvis Face: bilateral coxitis

FOGD showed a mosaic appearance and biopsy objectified partial villous atrophy.

Abdominal ultrasound showed splenomegaly and dilatation of the splenic vein and portal vein.

In _total_:

> Certain celiac disease put on GFD, martial therapy and vitamin D calcium supplementation.

> Seropositive and destructive rheumatoid arthritis put on corticosteroids minibolus for 3 days relayed by 10 mg of prednisone per day. Methotrexate-based background treatment at a dose of 15 mg/week was instituted after correction of the

hepatic balance.

> Autoimmune thyroiditis with fructal hyperthyroidism put on avlocardyl.

> For the hepatic involvement, a liver biopsy (LBP) was indicated but refused by the patient. The evolution was marked by a normalization of the hepatic balance under RSG.

OBSERVATIONS.

❖ Patient A.B aged 30 years, type 1 diabetic on insulin, with a history of mitro-aortic disease of rheumatic origin, a chronic anemia not improved by martial therapy, was hospitalized in our department for management of hypocalcemia at 1.1mmol/l.

On questioning, we find the sensation of paresthesias in both hands, the notion of chronic diarrhea with recent weight loss.

On clinical examination the chvostek sign was positive. The electrocardiogram - (ECG) showed a prolongation of the QT space. The ophthalmological examination revealed a bilateral subcapsular cataract.

Biologically, there was a microcytic iron deficiency anemia at 8.9g/dl associated with stigmata of malabsorption with low cholesterol and low PT at 35%. Hypocalcemia was confirmed at 1.1mmol/l with hyperphosphatemia at 2.2mmol/l. Biological myolysis was also present with creatine phosphokinase (CPK) at 40 times normal and lactate dehydrogenase (LDH) at 10 times normal.

The parathotmone (PTH) assay was down to 2.1pg/ml.

Muscle testing was normal with a normal electromyogram (EMG) and normal cardiac enzymes.

In view of this anemia with weight loss and the notion of diarrhea, a celiac disease serology was requested.

Anti-gliadin IgA positive at 92U/ml, anti-gliadin IgG positive at 81U/ml and anti-endomysium IgA positive.

The FOGD showed a mosaic aspect and the biopsy objectified a subtotal villous atrophy allowing to retain the diagnosis of celiac disease.

In total:

30-year-old adult male who presents:

❖ type 1 diabetes on insulin

❖ a definite celiac disease on GFD

❖ idiopathic hypoparathyroidism on Calperos® and un-alfa®.

❖ CPK elevation with a negative etiological investigation, corrected after the correction of the calcemia.

3.2 Comparison between celiac patients with and without associated autoimmune disease

The analysis of some parameters in our patients with and without associated diseases allowed us to conclude that only the presence of positive NAAs was significantly correlated with the presence of a pathology associated with celiac disease (p=0.038) (Table III).

Table III: Influence of the presence of an associated disease on the parameters of celiac disease

	Patients without associated diseases (n=25)	*Patients with associated diseases (n=18)*	*P*
Average age (years) + standard deviation	27,8 ±12,4	29,11 ±9,2	0,65
Female (n) (%)	22 (88%)	17 (94,4 %)	0,47
General signs	19	12	0,4
Weight loss	15	13	0,75
Chronic diarrhea	16	13	0,64
Osteomalacia	5	5	0,55
Recurrent oral aphthosis	4	0	8,098
Hypoalbuminemia	3	5	0,17
Hypergammaglobulinemia	4	13	0,41
IgA Transglutaminase positive (n)	18	12	0,25

IgA gliadin positive	8	3	0,3
IgG gliadin positive	7	5	0,41
Positive NAA (n)	4	9	**8,038**
Total villous atrophy	9	3	0,13

4. Discussion

4.1. Type 1 diabetes and celiac disease

❖ The association between celiac disease and type 1 diabetes has long been recognized. These two autoimmune diseases have genetic similarities through association with the DQ 2 region of the HLA class II major histocompatibility complex but also both diseases share non-HLA dependent loci [6,7].

❖ The prevalence of CD is 4 to 6 times higher in adults with type 1 diabetes than in the general population.

It has been shown in several studies that CD is more common in children with type 1 diabetes, but recent genetic and epidemiological studies and screening data suggest that CD has a high prevalence in adults with type 1 diabetes and the prevalence is estimated to be between 3.8 and 6.4% at diagnosis and the frequency of asymptomatic forms varies between 35 and 67% [8,9,10,11].

❖ For children, the International Diabetes Federation recommends routine screening for CD at diagnosis and then every year for 5 years [12]. Screening for CD in adults with diabetes varies according to the recommendations.

For the American College of Gastroenterology, the search for CD in type 1 diabetics is only suggested in case of digestive or extra digestive clinical signs or biological abnormalities [13].

According to NICE recommendations, serological testing for CD is indicated at the time of diagnosis of type 1 diabetes [14]

In our series, type 1 diabetes was found in 4 cases (9.3%).

4.2. Autoimmune thyroiditis

❖ The association between CD and Hashimoto's thyroiditis is widely studied. Hashimoto's thyroiditis was the most common disorder in association with CD according to a retrospective study done by Bibbo et al in 2017 that collated 255 known celiac patients and 250 controls over a 4-year period and aimed to determine the prevalence of IAD.

The frequency of thyroiditis was estimated at 24.3% with a significant difference compared to the healthy population (10%), followed by psoriasis with an estimated prevalence of 4.3%, then type 1 diabetes and Sjögren's syndrome with frequencies of 2.7 and 2.4% respectively, again with a significant difference [15].

❖ Sategna et al investigated the prevalence of dysthyroidism and particularly autoimmune thyroiditis in 241 celiacs and 212 controls. The prevalence of AIT was estimated at 16.2% (3.8% for controls) with a significant difference [16].

❖ A meta-analysis that studied series of patients with autoimmune thyroiditis in which the prevalence of AD and in particular CD was investigated, confirms this association [17].

❖   Thus, and according to NICE recommendations, serological testing for CD is indicated at the time of diagnosis of autoimmune thyroiditis [14].

In our series, thyroiditis with positive antithyroid antibodies was associated with CD in 4 cases or 9.3%. Hypothyroidism was found in 5 cases (11.6%) but antithyroid antibodies were requested in only one case.

4.3. Sjögren's syndrome

❖   Sjögren's syndrome (SS) is a connectivity that has been described by several authors in association with CD.

The involvement of gluten as a risk factor for autoimmune diseases is a matter of debate, but finally the results of several studies comparing the occurrence of IDA on a gluten-free and a gluten-free diet were not univocal [18,19].

❖   In the study by Bibbo et al, the frequency of SS in celiac patients was 2.4% compared to the healthy population (frequency of 0.4%), and this association was significant (p<0.0001) [15].

4.4. Systemic lupus erythematosus and celiac disease

❖   Since the 1980s, case series have indicated a possible association between these two diseases [20,21,22,23,24,25] but population-based studies are lacking.

❖   To further investigate this association, Ludvigsson et al compared the risk of SLE in 29,048 individuals with biopsy-verified CD (Marsh stage 3 villous atrophy) collected from 28 pathology departments in Sweden with 144,352 matched individuals from the general population identified by the Swedish total population registry [26]. The collected SLE cases were defined in the Swedish national patient registry. During follow-up, 54 individuals with CD developed SLE, a 3.5-fold increase in risk compared with the population. After 5 years of follow-up, the occurrence of SLE was 2.54 times more frequent [26].

❖ The association of these two diseases is multifactorial, related to shared genetic risk factors, involvement of the innate immune system, in particular Toll-like receptors (TLRs), as well as several common cytokine and chemokine pathways including interleukin 21.

Many HLA and non-HLA risk genes are shared between CD and SLE. Ninety percent of CD patients carry the DQ2 allele, which is often present with the DR3 haplotype, and two-thirds of patients with SLE carry the DR2 or DR3 haplotype [27].

❖ In our study, SLE was found in 3 cases (6.9%), this frequent association can be explained by the selection bias.

4.5. Rheumatoid arthritis

Rheumatoid arthritis and celiac disease are two separate entities that differ in their HLA predispositions and their specific predictive and diagnostic biomarkers. However, they share several aspects.

❖ Epidemiologically, they share a female predominance, environmental influences of comparable incidence, and associated antibodies.

❖   Clinically, celiac disease has both extraintestinal and gastrointestinal rheumatic manifestations. Small bowel pathology exists in rheumatic patients.

❖   Pathophysiologically, both diseases are mediated by endogenous enzymes in the target organs. Infectious, dysbiotic, and increased intestinal permeability theories as factors in the autoimmune cascade apply to both diseases [28].

❖   In contrast to their HLA-specific predisposition, the diseases share several non-HLA loci. These genes are crucial for the activation and regulation of innate and adaptive immunity [29].

❖   Two cases of rheumatoid arthritis were associated with CD in our series.

4.6. Primary biliary cirrhosis

❖   The association of CD and primary biliary cirrhosis (PBC) was reported by Logan et al in 1978 [30].

Subsequently, this association has been extensively studied by screening for CD in known PBC patients. The reported prevalence of CD during PBC varies considerably between studies (0% to 11%) and the average is 2.7% [31,32,33,34].

❖   Two large Swedish and English studies strongly support an association between CD and PBC. The Swedish cohort study including 8631 patients with CD found that the prevalence of PBC in these patients is increased by at least 20-fold compared with the normal population [35]. The second English study of 4732 subjects with CD and 23,620 age- and sex-matched subjects showed that the prevalence of PBC was 0.17% in patients with CD versus 0.05% in controls (3-fold increase) [36].

❖ It should be noted that "seronegative" forms of PBC (without anti-mitochondrial antibodies) associated with CD have been described [37].

❖ It has been suggested that PBC is promoted by increased intestinal permeability due to CD, which results in exposure of the immune system and liver to potential antigenic triggers including some microbial antigens

[37] . Furthermore, PBC and CD are thought to share the same predisposing terrain for autoimmunity, as reflected by the frequent association (53% of cases) of PBC with other autoimmune diseases (scleroderma, autoimmune thyroiditis, or Sjögren's syndrome).

❖ No cases of PBC were found in our series.

4.7. Autoimmune hepatitis

❖ The small number of reported cases of CD-autoimmune hepatitis (HAI) in the literature does not support a primary link between the two conditions.

❖ Two studies showed that the prevalence of CD in patients with HAI was 4% to 6.4%. Celiac disease was found in both types of HAI. Although intestinal biopsy showed histologic evidence of CD in addition to immunology, few cases had digestive symptoms [38,39].

❖ Both diseases are associated with HLA class II molecules encoded by HLA complex genes on chromosome 6, a region in which many autoimmune diseases are linked to specific alleles or combinations of alleles (haplotypes).

CD is associated with the HLA-DQ2 or HLA-DQ8 haplotype, whereas HAI is associated with HLA-DR3, HLA-DR4 or HLADR52 [40,41]. This HLA- B8DR3 region is closely related to HLA-DQ2 which could explain the association between the two diseases.

❖ Only one case of HAI was found in our series.

4.8. Selective IgA deficiency

❖ Selective IgA deficiency is the most common primary immune deficiency. Its biological definition is a profound decrease in IgA levels without alteration of IgG, IgM, IgE or IgG subclasses. Most of the time, it is only a case of a person without any particular symptom and in whom the dosage has been done in the framework of a general check-up. It is therefore most often an abnormality without any real pathology of the immune system.

IgA deficiency may cause an increased susceptibility to infections.

❖ The origin of IgA deficiency is still completely mysterious at the present time.

Associations with autoimmune diseases have been described and can occur throughout the life of patients (rheumatoid arthritis, SLE, immunological thrombocytopenic purpura...).

❖ IgA deficiency is more common in patients with CD (2-3%) than in the general population (1/400 to 1/800) [42,43].

❖ Della Libera et al tried to verify this association in a pediatric setting, in a cohort of 6625 patients, they measured IgA levels which were low in 50 cases. Celiac disease serology was performed for these patients and definite celiac disease confirmed by duodenal biopsy was found in 23% of patients [44].

❖ Because of the low circulating IgA level, screening for celiac disease by IgA-based serologic tests is not possible and it is therefore recommended that total IgA be routinely assayed in any patient suspected of having celiac disease in search of IgA deficiency, predisposing to this condition.

If IgA deficiency is present, it is currently recommended to assay anti-deamidated gliadin IgG and anti-transglutaminase IgG [13,45,46].

❖ Conversely, the association of a variable common immune deficiency (VCID) with celiac disease is exceptional.

The distinction between hypogammaglobulinemia secondary to digestive malabsorption and malabsorption syndrome occurring in the context of CVID is not always easy and it is the notion of recurrent airway infections, evolving for several years, that supports the diagnosis of CVID [47].

The malabsorption syndrome specific to CVID is due to a villous atrophy, most often incomplete, associated with a lymphocytic infiltration of the lamina propria considered as primitive, insensitive to the gluten-free diet and therefore different, by definition, from celiac disease [48,49].

❖ Selective IgA deficiency was found in 1 patient (2.3%) and CVID in 2 patients, one of whom was already being followed in the hematology department and was taking immunoglobulins on a regular basis.

4.9. Immunologic thrombocytopenic purpura

❖ Immunologic thrombocytopenic purpura (ITP) is an autoimmune disorder generated by the presence of anti-platelet autoantibodies [50].

❖ We have recently observed an increased prevalence of chronic autoimmune diseases in celiac patients and more specifically a tendency to polyautoimmunity [15].

Particular attention has been paid to the association of CD with ITP through several reported cases [51,52,53,54,55,56,57,58].

❖ A large study was done in 2008 by Olen et al.

This involved a cohort of 14 347 individuals with a hospital diagnosis of CD and 69

967 reference individuals matched for age, sex, and geographic region obtained from

the Swedish National Inpatient Register.

This study concluded that there was a 3-fold increase in the risk of ITP in celiacs and

a 6-fold increase in the risk of CD in known ITPs [59].

❖ Two cases of ITP associated with CD were noted in our series, i.e., 4.6%, which

confirms the association between the 2 conditions.

5. Conclusion

Adult CD is often associated with other autoimmune diseases. Their systematic search allows to avoid any diagnostic and therapeutic delay with a better prognosis.

References

[1] **Marsh MN**.

Gluten, major histocompatibility complex, and the small intestine.

Gastroenterology, 1992, **102**, 330-354.

[2] **Gasbarrini G, Miele L, Corazza GR, Gasbarrini A.**

When was celiac disease born?

J Clin Gastroenterol 2010; 44:502-503.

[3] **Nion-Larmurier I, Cosnes J.**

Celiac disease.

Clinical and Biological Gastroenterology 2009; 33:508-517.

[4] **Green PH, Cellier C.**

Celiac disease. N Engl J Med 2007; 357:1731-43.

[5] Ludvigsson JF, Rubio-Tapia A, van Dyke CT, Melton LJ 3rd, Zinsmeister AR, Lahr BD, Murray JA.

Increasing incidence of celiac disease in a North American population.

Am J Gastroenterol. 2013;108(5):818-24.

[6] **Smyth DJ, Plagnol V, Walker NM, et al.**

Shared and distinct genetic variants in type 1 diabetes and celiac disease.

N Engl J Med 2008;359:2767e77

[7] Barker JM.

Clinical review: Type 1 diabetes-associated autoimmunity: Natural history, genetic associations, and screening.

J Clin Endocrinol Metab 2006;91: 1210e7.

[8] Vicuna Arregui M, Zozaya Urmeneta JM, Martinez de Esteban JP, et al.

Study of celiac disease in adults with type 1 diabetes mellitus.

Gastroenterol Hepatol 2010;33:6e11.

[9] Aygun C, Uraz S, Damci T, et al.

Celiac disease in an adult Turkish population with type 1 diabetes mellitus.

Dig Dis Sci 2005;50:1462e6.

[10] Remes-Troche JM, Rios-Vaca A, Ramirez-Iglesias MT, et al.

High prevalence of celiac disease in Mexican Mestizo adults with type 1 diabetes mellitus.

J Clin Gastroenterol 2008;42:460e5.

[11] Mahmud FH, Murray JA, Kudva YC, et al.

Celiac disease in type 1 diabetes mellitus in a North American community: Prevalence, serologic screening, and clinical features.

Mayo Clin Proc 2005;80:1429e34.

[12] **International Diabetes Federation.**

Other complications and associated conditions. Global IDF/ISPAD guidelines for diabetes in childhood and adolescence; 2011:124e8.

[13] **Rubio-Tapia A, Hill I. D, Kelly C. P, Calderwood A. H, Murray J. A.**

ACG Clinical Guidelines: Diagnosis and Management of Celiac Disease. The American

Journal of Gastroenterology 2013; 108(5), 656-676.

[14] **Downey L, Houten R, Murch S, Longson D.**

Recognition, assessment, and management of coeliac disease: summary of updated NICE guidance.

BMJ 2015;351:h4513.

[15] **Bibbo S, Pes G. M, Usai-Satta P, Salis R, Soro S, Quarta Colosso B. M, Dore M. P.**

Chronic autoimmune disorders are increased in coeliac disease.

Medicine 2017; 96(47), e8562.

[16] **Sategna-Guidetti C.**

Prevalence of thyroid disorders in untreated adult celiac disease patients and effect of gluten withdrawal: an Italian multicenter study.

The American Journal of Gastroenterology 2001; 96(3), 751-757.

[17] **Fallahi P, Ferrari S. M, Ruffilli I, Elia G, Biricotti M, Vita R et al.**

The association of other autoimmune diseases in patients with autoimmune thyroiditis: Review of the literature and report of a large series of patients.

Autoimmunity Reviews 2016; 15(12), 1125-1128.

[18] **Sategna Guidetti C, Solerio E, Scaglione N, et al.**

Duration of gluten exposure in adult coeliac disease does not correlate with the risk for autoimmune disorders.

Gut 2001;49:502-5.

[19] **Ventura A, Magazzu G, Greco L.**

Duration of exposure to gluten and risk for autoimmune disorders in patients with celiac disease. SIGEP Study Group for Autoimmune Disorders in Celiac Disease.

Gastroenterology 1999;117:297-303.

[20] **Mukamel M, Rosenbach Y, Zahavi I, Mimouni M, Dinari G.**

Celiac disease associated with systemic lupus erythematosus.

Isr J Med Sci 1994;30:656-8.

[21] **Komatireddy GR, Marshall JB, Aqel R, Spollen LE, Sharp GC.** Association of systemic lupus erythematosus and gluten enteropathy.

South Med J 1995;88:673-6.

[22] **Romano C, Bartolone S, Sferlazzas C, Larosa D, Magazzu G.**

Systemic lupus erythematosus and coeliac disease.

Clin Exp Rheumatol 1997;15:582-3.

[23] **Mirza N, Bonilla E, Phillips PE.**

Celiac disease in a patient with systemic lupus erythematosus: A case report and review of literature. Clin Rheumatol 2007;26:827-8.

[24] **Rensch MJ, Szyjkowski R, Shaffer RT, Fink S, Kopecky C, Grissmer L, et al.** The prevalence of celiac disease autoantibodies in patients with systemic lupus erythematosus.

Am J Gastroenterol 2001;96:1113-5.

[25] **Freeman HJ.**

Adult celiac disease followed by onset of systemic lupus erythematosus.

J Clin Gastroenterol 2008;42:252-5.

[26] **Ludvigsson JF, Rubio-Tapia A, Chowdhary V, Murray JA, Simard JF.**

Increased risk of systemic lupus erythematosus in 29,000 patients with biopsy-verified celiac disease. J Rheumatol 2012;39:1964-70.

[27] Graham RR, Ortmann W, Rodine P, Espe K, Langefeld C, Lange E, et al. Specific combinations of HLA-DR2 and DR3 class II haplotypes contribute graded risk for disease susceptibility and autoantibodies in human SLE.

Eur J Hum Genet 2007;15:823-30

[28] Lerner A., Matthias T.

Rheumatoid arthritis-celiac disease relationship: Joints get that gut feeling.

Autoimmunity Reviews 2015; 14(11), 1038-1047.

[29] Zhernakova A, Stahl E. A, Trynka G, Raychaudhuri S, Festen E. A, Franke L. et al.

Meta-Analysis of Genome-Wide Association Studies in Celiac Disease and Rheumatoid

Arthritis Identifies Fourteen Non-HLA Shared Loci.

PLoS Genetics 2011; 7(2), e1002004.

[30] Logan RF, Ferguson A, Finlayson ND, Weir DG.

Primary biliary cirrhosis and coeliac disease: an association?

Lancet 1978;1: 230-233.

[31] **31] Pollock DJ.**

The liver in celiac disease.

Histopathology 1997;1:421-430.

[32] **Green RM, Flamm S.**

AGA technical review on the evaluation of liver chemistry tests.

Gastroenterology 2002;123:1367-1384.

[33] **Gillett HR, Cauch-Dudek K, Jenny E, Heathcote EJ, Freeman HJ.**

Prevalence of IgA antibodies to endomysium and tissue transglutaminase in primary biliary cirrhosis.

Can J Gastroenterol 2000; 14:672-675.

[34] **Floreani A, Betterle C, Baragiotta A, Martini S, Venturi C, Basso D, et al.**

Prevalence of coeliac disease in primary biliary cirrhosis and of antimitochondrial antibodies in adult coeliac disease patients in Italy.

Dig Liver Dis. 2002;34:258-61.

[35] **Sorensen HT, Thulstrup AM, Blomqvist P, Norgaard B, Fonager K, Ekbom A.**

Risk of primary biliary liver cirrhosis in patients with celiac disease: Danish and Swedish cohort study.

Gut 1999;44:736-738. 39.

[36] **Lawson A, West J, Aithal GP, Logan RFA.**

Autoimmune cholestatic liver disease in people with celiac disease: a population-based study of their association.

Aliment Pharmacol Ther 2005;21:401-405.

[37] **Rubio-Tapia A, Murray JA.**

The liver in celiac disease.

Hepatology 2007; 46: 1650-8.

[38] **Volta U, DeFranceschi L, Molinaro N, Cassani F, Muratori L, Lenzi M, et al.** Frequency and significance of anti-gliadin and anti-endomysial antibodies in autoimmune hepatitis.

Dig Dis Sci 1998;43:2190-2195.

[39] **Villalta D, Girolami D, Bidoli E, Bizarro N, Tampoia M, Liguori M, et al.** High prevalence of celiac disease in autoimmune hepatitis detected by anti-tissue transglutaminase autoantibodies.

J Clin Lab Anal 2005;19:6- 10

[40] **Tollefsen S, Arentz-Hansen H, Fleckenstein B, Molberg O, Raki M, Kwok WW, et al.**

HLA-DQ2 and -DQ8 signatures of gluten T cell epitopes in celiac disease.

J Clin Invest 2006;116:2226-2236. 50.

[41] **Krawitt EL.**

Autoimmune hepatitis.

N Engl J Med 2006;354:54-66. 51.

[42] **Conrad K , Roggenbuck D , Ittenson A et al.**

A new dot immunoassay for simultaneous detection of celiac specifi c antibodies and IgA- deficiency .

Clin Chem Lab Med 2012; 50: 337 - 43 .

[43] **McGowan KE , Lyon ME , Butzner JD .**

Celiac disease and IgA defi ciency: complications of serological testing approaches encountered in the clinic . Clin Chem 2008 ; 54 : 1203- 9 .

[44] **Della Libera I, Martelossi S, Tommasini, A.**

Selective IgA Deficiency: Ruling out Coeliac Disease and Selective Antibody Deficiency to Polysaccharides.

Journal of Clinical Immunology2013; 33(7), 1149-1149.

[45] **Villalta D , Alessio MG , Tampoia M et al.**

Testing for IgG class antibodies in celiac disease patients with selective IgA deficiency. A comparison of the diagnostic accuracy of 9 IgG anti-tissue transglutaminase, 1 IgG antigliadin and 1 IgG anti-deaminated gliadin peptide antibody assays .

Clin Chim Acta 2007; 382: 95 - 9 .

[46] **Villalta D , Tonutti E , Prause C et al.**

IgG antibodies against deamidated gliadin peptides for diagnosis of celiac disease in patients with IgA deficiency .

Clin Chem 2010; 56: 464 - 8 .

[47] **Bloch-Michel C, Viallard JF, Blanco P, Liferman F, Neau D, Moreau JF, et al.**

Variable common immune deficiency in adults: a clinical, biological and immunological study in 17 patients.

Rev Med Interne 2003;24:640-50.

[48] **Green PH, Jabri B.**

Coeliac disease.

Lancet 2003;362:383-91.

[49] **Béchade D, Desramé J, De Fuentès G, Camparo P, Raynaud J, Algayres J.-P.**

Variable common immune deficiency and celiac disease.

Clinical and Biological Gastroenterology 2004; 28(10), 909-912.

[50] Cines DB, Blanchette VS.

Immune thrombocytopenic purpura.

The New England Journal of Medicine 2002; 346 (13): 995-1008.

[51] Sheehan NJ, Stanton-King K.

Polyautoimmunity in a young woman.

Rheumatology 1993; 32 (3): 254-256.

[52] Kahn O, Fiel MI, Janowitz HD.

Celiac sprue, idiopathic thrombocytopenic purpura, and hepatic granulomatous disease: an autoimmune linkage?

Journal of Clinical Gastroenterology 1996; 23 (3): 214-216.

[53] Sarbay H, Cosan Sarbay B, Akin M, Kocamaz H, Tosun MS.

Celiac disease presenting with immune thrombocytopenic purpura.

Case Rep Hematol. 2017;2017:6341321.

[54] Roganovic J.

Celiac disease with Evans syndrome and isolated immune thrombocytopenia in monozygotic twins: a rare association.

Seminars in Hematology 2016; 53: S61-S63.

[55] Dogan M, Sal E, Akbayram S, Peker E, Cesur Y, Oner AF.

Concurrent celiac disease, idiopathic thrombocytopenic purpura and autoimmunethyroiditis: a case report.

Clin Appl Thromb Hemost. 2011;17(6):E13-6.

[56] Yamout B, Usta J, Itani S, Yaghi S.

Celiac disease, Behçet, and idiopathic thrombocytopenic purpura in siblings of a patient with multiple sclerosis.

Mult Scler. 2009;15(11):1368-71.

[57] Altintas A1, Pasa S, Cil T, Bayan K, Gokalp D, Ayyildiz O.

Thyroid and celiac diseases autoantibodies in patients with adult chronic idiopathicthrombocy topenic purpura.

Platelets. 2008;19(4):252-7.

[58] Williams SF, Mincey BA, Calamia KT.

Inclusion body myositis associated with celiac sprue and idiopathic thrombocytopenicpurpura

South Med J. 2003;96(7):721-3.

[59] **Olén O, Montgomery SM, Elinder G, Ekbom A, Ludvigsson JF.**

Increased risk of immune thrombocytopenic purpura among inpatients with coeliacdisease.

Scand J Gastroenterol. 2008;43(4):416-22.

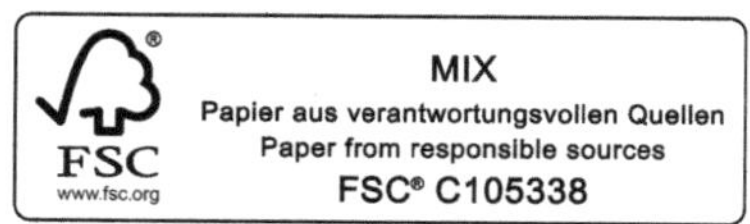

Printed by Books on Demand GmbH, Norderstedt / Germany